PATIENT'S MANUAL FOR CBASP

PATIENT'S MANUAL FOR
FOR
CBASP

James P. McCullough, Jr., PhD

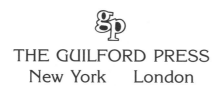

THE GUILFORD PRESS
New York   London

© 2003 James P. McCullough, Jr.
Published by The Guilford Press
A Division of Guilford Publications, Inc.
72 Spring Street, New York, NY 10012
www.guilford.com

Printed in the United States of America

This book is printed on acid-free paper.

Last digit is print number: 9   8   7   6   5   4   3   2   1

Library of Congress Cataloging-in-Publication Data

McCullough, James P.
  Patient's manual for CBASP / James P. McCullough, Jr.
    p. cm.
  ISBN 1-57230-814-1
    1. Depression, Mental—Popular works.   2. Cognitive therapy—Popular
works.   I. Title: Cognitive behavioral analysis system of
psychotherapy.   II. Title: CBASP.   III. Title.
RC537 .M3929 2003
616.85'270651—dc21

2002012527

To the millions of chronically depressed adults who, with some help, can experience an exodus from captivity.

About the Author

James P. McCullough, Jr., received his PhD from the University of Georgia in 1970. He is a fellow in two divisions (Psychotherapy and Clinical Psychology) of the American Psychological Association. Dr. McCullough was also elected a Diplomate in Clinical Psychology by the American Board of Psychological Forensic Examiners and is director of the Adult Psychotherapy Process Track in the Clinical Training Program at Virginia Commonwealth University (VCU) in Richmond. Currently a Professor of Psychology and Psychiatry and a member of VCU's graduate faculty, he has served since 1972 in the VCU Department of Psychology, where his colleagues gave him the award for Distinguished Research Contribution in Psychology in 2000. Teaching psychotherapy to clinical psychology graduate students has been his overarching educational contribution for the past three decades.

Strongly advocating single-case clinical research that emerges out of practice, Dr. McCullough developed a psychotherapy model, the Cognitive Behavioral Analysis System of Psychotherapy, out of his treatment of chronically depressed outpatients. He is the author of many publications, including *Treatment for Chronic Depression: Cognitive Behavioral Analysis System of Psychotherapy* and *Skills Training Manual for Diagnosing and Treating Chronic Depression: Cognitive Behavioral Analysis System of Psychotherapy*. He founded the Unipolar Mood Disorders Institute at VCU in 1992.

Preface

This manual was written to prepare you for CBASP psychotherapy. We want you to have a successful experience. We also feel strongly that the more you know about what you will be doing, the more positive your treatment outcome will be.

Please try to read the manual before your next therapy session. Take your time and don't worry about accomplishing all the things that you are going to read about. Remember, you are reading this manual without the company of the trained CBASP guide who, once you begin CBASP treatment, will "walk" with you, teach you the skills you'll need to overthrow your depression, and enthusiastically support and encourage your efforts.

Read the manual with the thought in mind that we are trying to impart hope to you right now, when you need it most. We are hopeful for you as you begin treatment. CBASP is designed to help patients who have the kinds of problems you are experiencing.

We also want to encourage you to reread this manual from time to time during your treatment. Write down any questions you have about the manual and discuss them with your therapist.

Best wishes to you as you begin CBASP treatment!

JAMES P. MCCULLOUGH, JR., PHD
Professor of Psychology and Psychiatry
Virginia Commonwealth University

Contents

PART I

THE CHRONICALLY DEPRESSED PATIENT

ONE

Introduction to the CBASP Manual

The CBASP *Patient Manual* was written especially for you and other people like yourself who suffer from chronic depression. Chronic depression is a biological and psychological disorder that lasts for two years or more; however, more often than not, our patients report being depressed for longer than 20 years. The purpose of this manual is to offer you hope as you enter CBASP psychotherapy. Chronic depression makes patients feel hopeless about ever living normally. With CBASP treatment, you will discover that your situation is not as hopeless as you think. Surprised? Don't be. Your CBASP therapist will show you what we mean by this assertion and why we say it to you.

Chronic depression has a way of negating all feelings of adequacy. Because nothing you have tried to do has decreased your symptoms, it is no wonder that you feel helpless and hopeless—both of which are prominent signs of the disorder. Your training in CBASP is going to equip you with effective coping skills and produce positive interpersonal experiences in your life, and these will help you overcome your feelings of helplessness and hopelessness.

We have great respect for the problems you face and the symptoms you experience. Depression is a formidable enemy. We know only too well how your depressive symptoms have undermined your sense of competence, self-confidence, and self-esteem. We also know that you are not likely to feel optimistic until you actually experience a decrease in symptoms, so it's fine with us if you remain skeptical about our treatment program. Just don't withdraw from treatment before you see what it can do for you.

Our major purpose in this manual is to share with you our optimism about your situation and to give you a brief look at how CBASP deals with chronic depressive disorder. Imagine this scenario, which describes an experience you've probably had at some point in your life.

> You've been sick, so you've gone to your doctor, not knowing what's wrong. Did you feel somewhat uneasy about your doctor's ability to help you get well? Maybe you were even worried that you had something really serious that might not have a cure. Did your doctor listen to you describe your symptoms, examine you, and then say something like this: "You have X, and here's what I want to do to treat it. You should be feeling better in a few days." Remember the relief and hope you felt at that moment?

Well, that is what we want you to feel now—relief and hope. Your depression is not untreatable, nor does it have to be a permanent condition. We have studied and treated chronic depression for over 20 years, and we have seen hundreds of people like yourself achieve normal and fulfilling lives. To reach the goal of feeling normal and fulfilled, however, requires hard work. We can guarantee you that your treatment experience will not be easy. You will have to commit yourself to working hard, both in and outside of your therapy sessions, by regularly completing your homework assignments, practicing and mastering the coping skills we teach you, and applying these newly learned skills in your daily life. Rest assured that your therapist will help you accomplish all of these goals every step of the way.

CBASP is specifically designed to treat the kind of depression you have by addressing the particular problems you have brought to treatment. You may be inclined to say:

> "Hey, wait a minute! You don't even know me, let alone what my problems are! How can you be so sure that CBASP will help me?"

The answer is, there are very *common problems* involved in all cases of chronic depression, and it is these common problems that CBASP is designed to remedy. However, even though we approach your chronic depression in a standardized way, you will be surprised to experience how we can still do justice to your uniqueness as a person as well as your life situation. In medicine, there are highly common features in any disease (for example, tuberculosis and tonsillitis) even though each human body is unique. These similar features usually make it possible to treat most diseases with one standardized procedure. Chronic depression is no exception. Rather than ignoring your unique circumstances, CBASP will help you deal with them in highly specific ways.

TWO

Two Types
of Chronic Depression

Your diagnosis of chronic depression means that you have been depressed for two years or more. Most patients who read this manual will have been depressed for a lot longer. The disorder involves both biological as well as psychological problems. Only the psychological issues of chronic depression and its treatment are discussed here. However, adequate treatment requires that you receive antidepressant medication in conjunction with CBASP psychotherapy. Your pharmacotherapist will discuss the biological issues of the disorder with you when you meet with him or her.

Chronic depression begins either during your childhood or adolescence ("early-onset chronic depression," which begins before age 21) or in adulthood, usually in the mid-20s ("late-onset chronic depression," which begins after age 20). Of course, there are exceptions to when depression begins among late-onset patients, but the majority of these patients report that their depression began before their 30th birthday. Depressive symptoms in both types vary in intensity over time. This means that sometimes your symptoms are more severe than at other times. Sometimes the symptoms mysteriously improve—even though they never fully disappear. When the more severe downward cycles occur, feelings of helplessness and hopelessness abound. The effects of these cycles are reminders that you have little or no control over how you feel. In the coming weeks, your CBASP therapist will help you understand *what* has been happening to you during the course of your chronic depression and *why*.

EARLY-ONSET CHRONIC DEPRESSION

If your depression onset began during childhood or adolescence, you will probably describe a family life that was difficult, to put it mildly. You may even use much stronger language to describe what it was like growing up in your family. It might have been filled with considerable stress, unhappiness, and interpersonal discord between you and your parent(s), siblings, or other family members. Your emotional trauma might have come from mistreatment by alcoholic parent(s), or you may have experienced physical abuse, sexual abuse, or grown up in a family where no one cared what you did, where you were, or when you came home. Some of our early-onset patients tell us that things were so bad in their homes that all they could do was try to "survive the hell of the family." Several case examples of early maltreatment and abuse are provided below.

CASE 1

"One of the earliest memories I have is being fondled by my father while he was bathing me in the tub. Sexual contact usually occurred when he had been drinking. During adolescence, I learned to stay away from him when he was drinking. Sometimes I couldn't avoid him, and his sexual advances occurred in spite of my protests."

CASE 2

"My mother beat me whenever I misbehaved or talked back to her. She would hit me with a stick or with her hand. She also told me that I was no good and that I would never amount to anything when I grew up. When I began to date, she frequently called me a 'whore' or a 'slut.' She kept trying to convince me that I was trash. I don't think I tried very hard to prove her wrong. Her abuse continued until I was 19 and moved out of the house. I haven't seen my mother in 10 years."

CASE 3

"Neither parent really loved me. My father worked all the time, and my mother was busy with her social life in the country club. She hung out at the club all the time. When I started driving, I used to stay out all night. They didn't care. No one cared. It's a miracle I didn't end up in jail or get in serious trouble. I wouldn't know what it feels like for someone to care for me."

LATE-ONSET CHRONIC DEPRESSION

If your depression onset began after age 20, then you fit into the late-onset group. More often than not, late-onset patients describe their growing-up years in less severe terms than do patients with early-onset beginnings. For example, they often recall one or more significant people whom they found to be helpful, loving, nurturing, and who enjoyed having them around. We also have found that the quality of the relationship patients have with their fathers appears to be better among late-onset patients than among those in the early-onset group. This is not to say that the family life of most late-onset patients was never difficult—not at all! Rather, it is to say that late-onset patients usually describe their early home environments as being less disruptive and not as conflict-filled as the environments described by most early-onset patients. Do any of these case examples sound familiar?

CASE 1

"I became depressed when I was 29 years old. That was nine years ago. My company was downsizing, and I found myself out of a job—very sudden and without any warning. Soon after that, my mother died suddenly. Then my wife and I began to have serious behavior problems with our two children. Both of our kids were in elementary school at the time. We couldn't agree on how to handle the problems, and we ended up arguing a lot. It took me about 18 months to find another job, and I've never really liked working for this company. It just seemed that my life turned sour nine years ago, and things have never gotten any better. Doesn't matter what I do, I stay depressed all the time."

CASE 2

"When I separated from my wife, I started feeling tired all the time. I had headaches, and I started missing a lot of work. I went to see my doctor and after I had described my symptoms, she told me I was depressed. She even gave me some kind of short test that she said confirmed that I was depressed. I took four or five different antidepressant medications over a period of three years, but nothing worked. I finally gave up, and I haven't taken any medicine for four years. I just stay down all the time, and I can't seem to shake it. This depression is messing up my life. I don't even feel like dating or going out with my friends. I have just about withdrawn from everything."

CASE 3

"I can't make myself do anything since my father died. He and I were real close, and when he died, nothing seemed very important to me anymore. He died almost seven years ago. I've tried to make myself go on, but it's no use, I just come home from work and go to sleep. I wake up the next morning and go back to work, starting the routine all over again. My friends urge me to see a psychiatrist and get on some kind of medicine, but I don't believe in that sort of thing. I've come to see you because I'm near the end of my rope. I can't go on like this. Life is not worth living anymore. I'm thinking more and more about ending it, and my thoughts about suicide have really frightened me."

The good news is that CBASP therapy is designed to treat both early- and late-onset types of chronic depression. Whether you are an early- or late-onset patient, you are a good candidate for CBASP therapy.

THREE

Common Problems of the Chronically Depressed Patient

We have noted that chronic depression leaves you extremely demoralized and feeling victimized by emotions you are unable to control—such as helplessness and hopelessness. *These responses of feeling helpless and hopeless stem, in part, from daily problems that you encounter and are unable to resolve.* It is no accident that a central goal of CBASP treatment is to teach you how to become a better problem solver. We don't want your daily problems to remain unresolved!

At the beginning of therapy, most of our patients are not very effective when it comes to solving their problems. In fact, they usually approach problem solving by engaging in two ineffective coping strategies. These negative strategies are described below. As you read the next few sections, see if your present thinking and behavior match our descriptions of the negative coping strategies of chronically depressed patients.

THE GLOBAL THINKING APPROACH TO COPING

The first ineffective approach to problem solving becomes evident when patients begin to talk about their problems with the therapist. They usually describe their problems in a global or overly general manner. The way they talk about their problems is illustrated in the following descriptions.

"Nothing will ever work out for me."
"No one could ever love or care for me."
"I'll always fail, no matter how hard I try."
"I feel like I'm a worthless person."
"People always end up rejecting me."
"This is just another example of how I always mess things up."
"It does no good to try because I'll just foul up things."
"My life is nothing but one disaster after another."
"People are never sensitive to my needs."
"I always feel used by others."
"People run over me all the time."
" 'Born to Lose' is my theme song."
"I knew my boss would not like what I did—no one ever has."
"I'll never have a good relationship with anyone."
"I'll always be incompetent."
"I can't do anything well."
"I'll never be able to learn this therapy stuff—I'll just fail again."
"Everyone thinks I'm stupid, that I can never do anything right."

Do any of these statements resemble the way you think and talk about your problems? Do you make any comments like these when things don't go your way or when you encounter a difficult situation with another person? If you answered "yes" to one or both of these questions, then you are thinking and talking in a global and overly general manner.

Most patients we see in CBASP therapy begin treatment talking about their problems in this way. Global approaches to problem solving *never* work—they are 100% guaranteed to fail. Why? When you think about your problems from a global perspective, you do not direct your energy toward any one problem in particular. Rather, the focus is on a general category of problems or problems-in-general. The problem-at-hand (the one causing the difficulty) is never addressed specifically. Problem resolution requires a specific plan of action; the problem-at-hand must be tackled directly. Now let's look at a second coping strategy that doesn't work.

THE "NOTHING I DO MATTERS" DEFEATIST APPROACH TO COPING

The second way chronically depressed patients approach problem solving is closely related to global thinking. In fact, this approach is a consequence or result of global thinking. It involves approaching a stressful situation by taking the "low road" and automatically concluding (as well as feeling):

> "Nothing I do matters, so why try?"
> "Even if I tried to change things and seek people out, I would end up at the same dead end—no one would like me."

This approach, like global thinking, *never* leads to problem resolution and *always* plunks you in the "loser's seat." Withdrawal or retreat from the stressful situation is likely to be the next step. Once again, the problem-at-hand is not addressed.

Global styles of defeatist thinking are the *big stoppers*, the *great self-destroyers*, that stand in the way of effective coping. They also leave patients in a perpetual state of despair. CBASP therapy will help you replace these negative approaches with a more effective, problem-focused style. As you become more skilled at problem solving, you will find that the feelings of helplessness and hopelessness begin to lessen.

CONSEQUENCES FOR GLOBAL/DEFEATIST THINKING

Whenever you think globally or retreat, in a defeatist way, from stressful situations, you are left feeling that your behavior is not important, that it really has no significant impact—no *consequences*. You are left in a "one-down" position with every problem you face. Things only get worse, never better, because your problems are never settled or resolved—they just stack up, one on top of the other, in a never ending pile. This pile-up of problems is why many patients, when they think about the future, see only more of the same old misery. Nothing can change as long as you approach living this way. It could even be said that as long as you think globally and assume that your actions don't matter, you have already written the end of your life story—and it ends in failure.

GOALS OF YOUR TREATMENT

CBASP therapy is designed to help you learn to behave differently. Specifically, it helps you *stop* approaching your problems from a global perspective, and it shows you that *everything* you do matters. Not only will you learn that your behavior has specific consequences for others (includ-

ing your therapist), you will also learn to recognize what these consequences are. You will even learn how to make choices about what kind of
consequences you *want* to have as well as learn the skills to produce what
you want. Sound incredible? It's really not. Once you begin to experience
your interpersonal power and realize that you now have the skills to use
that power effectively, the old feelings of helplessness and hopelessness
will fall away.

Now we must return to your current problems with chronic depression. We know that our description of the common problems that many
chronic patients face has not set you free. Nor will simply reading our
description of a better way to problem solve make you feel less depressed.
In therapy, however, you will learn how to change the way you live and
this change will lead to greater mood control.

The remainder of the *Patient Manual* introduces you to the CBASP
techniques that are designed to address the serious problems outlined in
this chapter.

PART II

AN INTRODUCTION TO CBASP TECHNIQUES

FOUR

Situational Analysis

DEALING WITH ONE PROBLEM AT A TIME

Since we cannot solve all your problems at once, we don't try. Instead, we take them one at a time, using a CBASP technique called *situational analysis*, or just "SA." SA counters global thinking by focusing on one "slice of time" when a particular problem occurred. SA also neutralizes the defeatist "what-I-do-doesn't-matter" approach to problem solving by requiring you to look at the consequences of your behavior: *You have to face the results of what you did during a period of time when you had a problem with your mate, a friend, boss, or business associate.* With SA, you learn quickly how you personally influence situations to come out the way they do. If you don't like the way a situation came out, then we'll help you revise what you did so that a more desirable outcome can be achieved the next time. We'll help you learn how *not* to make the same mistake again.

You may be thinking to yourself (and we hope you are):

"How will solving one problem at a time help me cure my chronic depression?"

You may not believe this the first time we say it, but we have found that most patients have problems with other people, and these problems fall into, at most, a very limited number of categories. Once patients straighten out these limited problem areas, they begin to report successful interpersonal encounters across a variety of situations. Once patients taste the thrill of success, symptoms begin to decrease. It's hard to remain depressed when you feel in control of your life and know that you can cope effectively with your problems.

You will experience several outcome benefits from learning to do SA:

1. *Action*: SA will focus your attention on a specific problem that occurs at a particular time and place.
   Outcome: Your global thinking will be countered and replaced with a more focused perspective.
2. *Action*: SA will teach you how to identify the effects (consequences) you have on other people.
   Outcome: Your defeatist "it-doesn't-matter-what-I-do" thinking will be neutralized and extinguished.
3. *Action*: SA will show you that you are interpersonally connected to the world you live in.
   Outcome: Learning that your behavior has consequences will produce a sense of empowerment in you.
4. *Action*: SA will expose the interpersonal problem behaviors that cause you to have difficulties with others.
   Outcome: We will help you remedy your interpersonal problems with behavioral skill training.
5. *Action*: SA will teach you to become a goal-oriented thinker.
   Outcome: You will learn to think about situational goals at the *beginning* of encounters with others, not *after* the fact.

There are other outcome benefits to doing SA, but these are some of the more important ones. Now we will shift gears and discuss two case examples to illustrate how SA rectifies global thinking and the defeatist "it-doesn't-matter-what-I-do" approach to problem solving.

TWO CASE EXAMPLES

Case 1: Mary

Mary is a 31-year-old divorced woman who has been depressed since she was 12 years old (early-onset). She has a 14-month-old son. On several occasions, usually following the breakup of a love affair, Mary's depression has become more severe. The last serious episode occurred two years ago, following her separation and divorce. During the past six months, however, Mary has felt only moderately depressed but says that she never really feels "good." She has a hard time describing any one problem, and she doesn't see how talking about one problem at a time is going to help her feel better. Mary describes her problems this way:

> "People are just not sensitive to my needs, and I often feel used by others—they take advantage of me."

Her therapist asks her *when* was the last time she felt someone was not sensitive to her needs or used her in some way. Mary's answer becomes the jumping off point for doing her first SA. The therapist anchors Mary's global complaint in a *slice-of-time*: that is, the therapist asks her to locate the complaint in a specific time and place so that, together, they can examine the nature of her problems more closely.

MARY: It was last Tuesday at noon, when I was attempting to feed my son. He was in his high chair in the kitchen.

THERAPIST: Let's do an SA on the situation. The first thing I want you to do is describe the situation for me. *Tell me what happened.* Remember, the first step in SA is a situational description. The description must have a beginning in time, an ending, and a "story" in between.

The SA form, called the Coping Survey Questionnaire (CSQ), that Mary and her therapist used in situational analysis is illustrated below in the Case 1 Coping Survey Questionnaire. Refer to Mary's CSQ as we take you through her SA.

Elicitation Phase of SA

STEP 1: Describing the Situation

MARY: My son was in his high chair, and I was feeding him lunch. The doorbell rang. I stopped feeding him, left my son in the chair, and went to the front door. It was my next-door neighbor, who is pushy and aggressive. She said that she needed a cup of sugar for a cake she was baking. I told her that this was not a good time and asked her to come back. I opened the door and let her in. She mumbled something about this not taking long and then asked me where the sugar was. I pointed her to the sugar bin on the counter and went back to feeding my son. She got the sugar and left. I was frustrated, mad, and then I got depressed and thought to myself: "I've been screwed again."

COPING SURVEY QUESTIONNAIRE

Patient: <u>Mary</u>   Therapist: <u>Dr. Rowan</u>

Date of Situational Event: <u>6-17-90</u>   Date of Therapy Session: <u>6-19-90</u>

<u>Instructions:</u> Select one problematical event that has happened to you during the past week and describe it using the format below. Please try to fill out all parts of the questionnaire. Your therapist will assist you in reviewing this situational analysis during your next therapy session.

Situational Area: Spouse/Partner __ Children __ Extended Family __
             Work/School __ Social √

Step 1. Describe <u>what</u> happened:

Feeding son lunch. Doorbell rang. Stopped feeding, left son in chair. Neighbor wanted to borrow a cup of sugar. Told her this is not a good time. She insisted. Asked her to come back. Opened door, stepped back, she came in. She went into kitchen and got a cup of sugar. Then she left.

Step 2. Describe your interpretation of what happened (how did you "read" the situation?):

1. I like to answer the doorbell when it rings.

<u>Revisions</u>

Need to revise! ➤

2. ~~People are insensitive to my needs.~~
3. ~~I cannot control my life.~~

2. Don't want to interrupt feeding my son.
3. Must tell neighbor she must come back later.

Step 3. Describe what you did during the situation (what you said and how you said it):

<u>Add Assertion</u>

Tell the lady "No, come back."

Answered doorbell. Told her this is not a good time. Asked her to come back. Held door open and let neighbor in. Pointed her to the sugar bin. Went back to feeding my son.

Step 4. Desribe how the event came out for your (actual outcome):

My son's lunch was interrupted when the neighbor came in.

Step 5. Desribe how you wanted the event to come out for you (desired outcome):

Wanted the neighbor to come back at a more convenient time.

Step 6. Was the desired outcome achieved?   YES ____   NO √

CASE 1. Mary's Coping Survey Questionnaire used for situational analysis.

STEP 2: Interpreting the Situation

THERAPIST: You've given us a good situational description. It has a clear beginning, a well laid-out story, and a clear ending point. Now, let's see what you put into this situation that influenced it to come out the way it did. The second step in SA involves your *interpretations* of the situation—that is, your understanding of *what* was taking place during this encounter. I want you to give me several interpretation sentences that state *what this situation means to you.*

MARY: (*after thinking several minutes*)
1. I like to answer the doorbell when it rings.
2. People are insensitive to my needs.
3. I cannot control my life.

Observe the global way Mary states her last two interpretations and also the "it-doesn't-matter-what-I-do" theme that emerges in them.

STEP 3: Describing the Situational Behavior

THERAPIST: You've given me three interpretation sentences. Now, the next step in SA is focusing on what you *did* in the situation. Try to answer this question: *What did you actually do in the situation? That is, how did you actually behave?*

MARY: Well, I went to the door and answered the doorbell. I even held the door open after telling the neighbor that this was not a good time and asking her to come back later. I pointed her to the sugar bin, and then I went back to feeding my son.

STEP 4: Pinpointing the Actual Outcome (AO)

THERAPIST: So now we see how you read the situation—your interpretations—and what you did during the event—your behavior. The next step in SA involves looking at how the situation *came out* for you. We call this the "actual outcome." *How did the event come out for you?*

MARY: My son's lunch was interrupted when the neighbor came in and got the sugar.

STEP 5: Pinpointing the Desired Outcome (DO)

THERAPIST: I've got the picture. The next question is an important one in that it involves something that didn't happen but might have, under different circumstances. *How would you have liked the situation to have come out for you?* We call this the "desired outcome."

MARY: I wanted her to come back at a more convenient time.

STEP 6: Comparing the Actual Outcome with the Desired Outcome

THERAPIST: Did you get what you wanted in this situation? That is, did the actual outcome equal the desired outcome?

MARY: No! Absolutely not! (*Mary got frustrated and angry at this point.*)

THERAPIST: Why didn't you get what you wanted here?

MARY: Because nothing ever works out for me, that's why! People take advantage of me because I'm a wimp. Nothing I want to do matters. My whole day was ruined by that stupid lady!

> *Do you see why Mary didn't obtain her desired outcome in the situation? The way Mary interpreted the situation—using global thinking and a "nothing-I-do-really-matters" approach—and then, how she behaved at the door while talking to the neighbor—saying "No" but then stepping back and holding the door open for her to enter—had a direct bearing on the way the situation ended. Of course, it's easy to be a "Monday morning quarterback" and see the right calls to make. In the heat of the game, it's much more difficult to call the right plays. Nevertheless, Mary paid a high price for the way she behaved in the situation. The price was her frustration, anger, and a ruined day. It takes just one or two ruined days to ruin a week, several bad weeks to ruin a month, and all of a sudden, life is out of control, and the person has a chronic depression on his or her hands.*

Situational problems look different under the SA microscope. At first they look harsh and impossible to resolve. However, most of the time these problems are fixable. We help you fix them during the remediation phase of SA, in which the therapist and patient systematically repair situational problems so that the desired outcome can be attained.

Remediation Phase of SA

After Mary's therapist explains the remediation procedure to her, her interpretations will be examined to determine if (1) they are global or anchored in the situation, and (2) to see if each interpretation accurately describes what happened between Mary and her neighbor, rather than falling into the "it-doesn't-matter-what-I-do" category; (3) lastly, the degree to which each interpretation contributed to the attainment of Mary's desired outcome is assessed.

STEP 1: Revising the Interpretations

THERAPIST: Mary, let's look at each interpretation. I'll ask you several questions about each one. First, is the interpretation anchored to the event? Second, does it accurately describe what happened between you and the neighbor? And third, how does your interpretation contribute to your obtaining what you want in the situation—that is, your desired outcome? If the interpretation is not anchored or if it doesn't accurately describe what took place, then we will have to *revise the interpretation* to meet these criteria. Interpretations cannot contribute to attaining your desired outcome unless they are anchored and accurate. There is something else about "contributory interpretations" that I will show you in a moment. Now, let's look at your first interpretation: "I like to answer the doorbell when it rings." Is this interpretation anchored and accurate, and did it contribute to your getting what you wanted in this situation?

MARY: Well, it's the way I feel but, no, it doesn't get me what I want.

THERAPIST: Yes, it's the way you feel, and it's clearly anchored to the beginning of the event and accurately describes what you want to do when the doorbell rings. It doesn't contribute to your desired outcome in this particular case, but at least you know where you are when the event begins. What about the adequacy of the second interpretation, "People are insensitive to my needs"? Is it anchored and accurate, and does it contribute to your getting the desired outcome?

MARY: No. It really has nothing to do with what is actually happening. I'm just thinking about people-in-general.

THERAPIST: So thinking globally about people-in-general won't get you what you want here. The interpretation doesn't contribute to obtaining the desired outcome or telling your neighbor to come back later. We've got to revise it so that it will help, not hinder, you in reaching your goal. Can you think of an anchored and accurate interpretation that does describe what actually went on here?

MARY: I don't want to interrupt feeding my son.

THERAPIST: Does this sentence express how you felt? If it does, then it's anchored and accurate and we can substitute it for the people-in-general interpretation.

MARY: It's how I feel as I look back at the situation.

THERAPIST: Look at your last interpretation: "I cannot control my life." Is this statement anchored and accurate, and does it contribute to getting the desired outcome?

MARY: It's like my second interpretation. It doesn't help me, and it's very global.

THERAPIST: You're right! It's not anchored, nor is it accurate. Let me describe one type of interpretation that you will need in this and many other situations you encounter. I call it an *action interpretation*. Action interpretations suggest what we must do or what assertive behaviors we must employ to obtain the desired outcome. They cut right to the heart of a situational problem and frequently help us resolve it. What if your third interpretation had been an action interpretation, like this?: "I've got to tell my neighbor that she must come back later because I'm feeding my son." Would this interpretation have contributed to your getting what you wanted—namely, for your neighbor to come back later?

MARY: It would have worked if I could have interpreted it that way. But I have trouble asserting myself to others.

STEP 2: Revising Situational Behavior

THERAPIST: You don't have to assert yourself right now. All we're trying to do is help you see the role interpretations play in successfully managing situations. Now, let me show you something about your first interpretation and the two revised ones. How would your situational behavior have changed if you had interpreted the situation with the revised interpretations, including the action interpretation?

MARY: I would have told her that she'd have to come back after I finished feeding my son, and I would not have held the door open for her to come in.

THERAPIST: Had you read the situation this way and behaved the way you just described, would you have gotten what you wanted?

MARY: Yes! I see what you are driving at here! I've got to change the way I interact with others in order to get what I want.

THERAPIST: You are right, and we'll keep working at it until you learn to achieve what you want.

Refer back to the Case 1 Coping Survey Questionnaire and review the therapist's notes in the margin of the CSQ to see how the situation looked once it had been "fixed." First, Mary's second and third interpretations had to be revised. Her global and inaccurate interpretations had to be "revised" and reconstructed before it would be possible for her to reach her goal. The way Mary interpreted the situation directly affected her behavior—which, until the interpretations were revised, made it impossible for her to achieve the desired outcome.

Most of Mary's problem-solving energies were not focused on the problem-at-hand but on "people-in-general" or on an "out-of-control life." With her attention anchored to the current event, she is in a position to take positive action. This brings us to the second change in the SA that had to be made in order for her to obtain the desired outcome: *her behavior.* Changing Mary's passive behavior into assertive behavior took a little time and practice, but it *was* accomplished, because now she understood that, more often than not, without assertive behavior she would not be able to obtain the desired outcome.

You may be thinking that assertion is fine and good but that you could never pull it off or say such things to a neighbor (especially to an aggressive and pushy neighbor). As noted above, Mary said the exact same thing to the therapist while her SA was being revised. Here's what the therapist said to Mary:

> "Mary, that's all right, you don't have to. But, when you're ready to resolve a problem like this one, you'll know what has to be done. Take your time. You'll get there."

The outcome of this case was a happy one. It didn't take Mary very long to begin asserting herself to others. Considering the possibility that she might actually become a problem solver was too attractive an alternative. When she tried out being assertive a few weeks later, she was surprised when she got what she wanted and by how much better she felt. There was no frustration, anger, or depression; instead, she was elated and proud of what she had accomplished.

Empowerment is the word CBASP therapists like to use to describe the results of this sort of interpersonal success. If you met Mary today, you would encounter a person who lets others know what she wants and doesn't want. She no longer feels that others are insensitive to her needs, nor does she feel used by people. Mary doesn't settle for this defeatist "loser perspective" anymore. It goes without saying that the old feelings of helplessness and hopelessness have faded. Her chronic depressive disorder has been in remission for 10 years.

Let's take one more case example to see how another CBASP patient used the Coping Survey Questionnaire to report a successfully managed situation. The patient, Ralph, describes an interpersonal situation in which he obtained his desired outcome.

Case 2: Ralph

Ralph is a 38-year-old accountant who has worked in the same large corporation for 17 years. He has been married for 14 years and has four children. He has done well if you measure "success" by the corporation's standards. This includes a string of positive evaluations over the last five years and a recent raise and promotion. The patient became depressed during his 24th year (late-onset), following an evaluation where he received a less-than-satisfactory rating in two work areas. His depression has never remitted; he has been depressed for 14 years. Ralph reported several episodes when he became severely depressed. One episode occurred eight years ago, when he was hospitalized for two weeks because of suicidal ideation. He has taken a number of medications over the years and is currently taking Paxil. The drug helps some, but no medication has cured the chronic depression. When Ralph talks about his problems, he describes them in global terms. He says things like the following:

"I'll always fail no matter how hard I try."
"I'll always be incompetent, because I can't do anything well."

Ralph's psychotherapist was surprised by these comments in light of his positive work record, a recent promotion, and consistent positive feedback from his work supervisor. He brought a completed Coping Survey Questionnaire to his 12th psychotherapy session. Ralph's questionnaire is shown in the Case 2 Coping Survey Questionnaire. Refer to it as we go through his SA.

COPING SURVEY QUESTIONNAIRE

Patient: Ralph   Therapist: Dr. Schultz

Date of Situational Event: 2-18-97   Date of Therapy Session: 2-22-97

Instructions: Select one problematical event that has happened to you during the past week and describe it using the format below. Please try to fill out all parts of the questionnaire. Your therapist will assist you in reviewing this situational analysis during your next therapy session.

Situational Area: Spouse/Partner √ Children __ Extended Family __
                   Work/School __ Social __

Step 1.   Describe <u>what</u> happened:

Told my wife I had appointment with you at the same time I was supposed to be home to meet our children when they came home from school. She reminded me of my oversight and got angry. I said I would not change our appointment, that I was sorry I forgot, but I would have to make other arrangements. She laid into me and called me a failure. I felt guilty, but I said I would get a babysitter. I did.

Step 2.   Describe your interpretation of what happened (how did you "read" the situation?):

     1.   I forgot all about our appointment and my agreement to be home.
     2.   I will not break the appointment with you.
     3.   Phyllis thinks I am a failure.
     4.   I've got to schedule a sitter to be here by 3:30 P.M. [action interpretation].

Step 3.   Describe what you did during the situation (what you said and how you said it):

     I listened to Phyllis. Told her I was sorry, but I wouldn't change appointment. Listened to her tell me I never carry my share of the family load. In matter-of-fact way, I said I would get sitter. I did.

Step 4.   Desribe how the event came out for your (actual outcome):

I got a sitter to be at our house by 3:30 P.M.

Step 5.   Desribe how you wanted the event to come out for you (desired outcome):

I wanted to get the sitter scheduled.

Step 6.   Was the desired outcome achieved?   YES √   NO ____

CASE 2. Ralph's Coping Survey Questionnaire used for situational analysis.

Elicitation Phase of SA

STEP 1: Describing the Situation

THERAPIST: Tell me what happened. I want you to give me a good idea of *when* the situation began and ended. Then tell me the story that happened between the two time points.

RALPH: Well, it had to do with the time of our appointment today. Last week we changed our regular appointment time to this hour. I'd forgotten that I told my wife that I would come home today and be there when the kids got home from school. The situation started last night. Phyllis and I were talking about our schedules, and I mentioned that I had an appointment with you at 3:00 P.M. She reminded me that I had said that I would be at home by 3:30 P.M. to meet the kids when they got home from school at 4:00. I told her that I didn't want to change our appointment—that I was really sorry that I'd forgotten, but that we would have to make other arrangements. She got furious. She told me that I never kept my word, that I was a failure, and that I didn't pull my share of the load around the house. I felt awful and started feeling really guilty. She wouldn't get off my case. I said again that I would not change the appointment but that I would get a sitter to be here by 3:30 P.M. She jumped up and stormed off to the bedroom. I called the sitter and worked out the schedule so that she would be here. Then I went to bed.

STEP 2: Interpreting the Situation

THERAPIST: This is a good situation to analyze, and I've got the general idea of what happened. Now, the next SA step has to do with your interpretations about what was going on. So, what did the event mean to you?

RALPH: (*looking down at the interpretations he had written*)
1. I forgot all about our appointment and my agreement to be home.
2. I will not break the appointment with you.
3. Phyllis thinks I am a failure.
4. I've got to schedule a sitter to be here by 3:30 P.M. [action interpretation].

STEP 3: Describing the Situational Behavior

THERAPIST: We've got four interpretations to work with. Now, tell me what you did in the situation. I mean, how did you behave with Phyllis during the event?

RALPH: I must have looked very surprised. I couldn't believe I'd forgotten our agreement. I listened to Phyllis for a long time, then told her, "I'm really sorry about this, but I won't change the appointment." I think I said this in a matter-of-fact way. This made her madder, but I wasn't going to change my mind. Finally, I told Phyllis that I would get a sitter, which I did. I don't think I raised my voice the entire time, but I felt awful and very guilty.

THERAPIST: So you didn't lose your cool, you apologized, and you told Phyllis that you would get a sitter to be at the house when the kids came home?

RALPH: Yes.

STEP 4: Pinpointing the Actual Outcome (AO)

THERAPIST: How did the event come out for you? What was the actual outcome?

RALPH: The event was a mess, a total disaster for Phyllis and me. But it ended up with my scheduling a sitter to be at the house today by 3:30 P.M.

STEP 5: Pinpointing the Desired Outcome (DO)

THERAPIST: How did you want the situation to come out? What was your desired outcome?

RALPH: I wanted to get the sitter scheduled.

STEP 6: Comparing the Actual Outcome with the Desired Outcome

THERAPIST: Did you get what you wanted here? That is, did the actual outcome match your desired outcome?

RALPH: Yes, it did.

THERAPIST: Why did it work out the way you wanted?

RALPH: Because I stayed focused. I remembered how we talked about the global and the "it-doesn't-matter-what-I-do" ways I usually approach my problems. I was determined not to lose my focus in this situation.

THERAPIST: I thought you did a fantastic job with this difficult situation! I'm not sure I could have done as well as you did.

RALPH: You know, I'm still surprised when you tell me that I do a good job. I keep expecting you to lay into me and tell me that I made a mistake and that I'm incompetent.

This is a difficult situation; even though Ralph obtained the desired outcome, the conflict with Phyllis still remains to be settled. You may be surprised to learn that therapists also must stay focused. In this situation, the
therapist must remain focused on Ralph's obvious success and not rush off
and try to settle the conflict with Phyllis. *Remember, only one problem can
be dealt with at a time!* Ralph has had an obvious success and, in the process, has learned some things about problem solving. Ralph's prognosis in
treatment looks very positive, based on how he applies what he learns in
the session to resolve his everyday problems. He also can utilize these
newly learned skills when he and Phyllis are ready to address their misun-
derstanding. Once you and I learn an effective way to solve problems,
then we can use the methodology everywhere. This is why CBASP
therapists don't have to solve all of an individual's problems. SA is a
problem-solving tool that can be applied anywhere, anytime. When
patients learn to apply SA to help them resolve problems in their daily
life, we call this step *transfer of learning.*

Remediation Phase of SA

When patients bring in successful SAs wherein they obtained the desired
outcome, we highlight and strengthen the interpretations and behaviors
that resulted in their success.

STEP 1: Highlighting the Successful Interpretations

THERAPIST: Let's go back and review your interpretations and see how
    they helped you get what you wanted. Was your first interpretation
    ["I forgot all about our appointment and my agreement to be home"]
    anchored and accurate?

RALPH: Yes. It was the truth, I totally forgot.

THERAPIST: What about the adequacy of the second interpretation ["I will
    not break the appointment with you"]?

RALPH: It was anchored and accurate.

THERAPIST: Was the third interpretation ["Phyllis thinks I'm a failure"]
    anchored and accurate?

RALPH: Yes. She told me as much, and it made me feel awful and guilty.

THERAPIST: What about the fourth interpretation ["I've got to schedule a
    sitter to be here by 3:30 P.M.]?

RALPH: I remembered about action interpretations, and I used one here. It

worked because it mobilized me to take immediate action and schedule the sitter.

THERAPIST: One more question. How did these four interpretations contribute to your getting what you wanted in this particular situation?

RALPH: The first thing that comes to mind is that they kept me grounded
and focused on the situation. I kept my "eye on the ball," so to speak.
I didn't get off into any side issues that would have taken me away
from the problem-at-hand.

STEP 2: Highlighting the Assertive Behavior

THERAPIST: Your interpretations led you to do what?

RALPH: As I said before, they mobilized me to fix the situation as best as I
could and to tell Phyllis what I was going to do. She didn't like it, but
at least she knew exactly what was going to happen.

Ralph's successful SA is quite different from Mary's. In Mary's case
(see Case 1 CSQ), the actual outcome did not match the desired outcome, so the therapist helped her fix the interpretations that created the
situational problems. As noted above, the therapist's strategy with Ralph
changed during the remediation phase; he had obtained what he wanted
because his interpretations were anchored and accurate and his behaviors
were task-appropriate (scheduling a sitter). We are also happy to report
that Ralph continues to counter his global thinking and the defeatist
"it-doesn't-matter-what-I-do" reactions with more problem-focused coping. Over time, he has used SA to demonstrate to himself that he is not a
failure, nor is he incompetent; rather, he is a successful employee, hus-
band, and father. Ralph has been without symptoms for two years.

Before we leave Ralph's case and go to Chapter 5, notice that Ralph's
SA performance on the Coping Survey Questionnaire met the prescribed
standards for each step. Ralph learned to do SA correctly by applying what
he learned in sessions to his homework assignments: He brought a completed CSQ to the session each week. At the outset, Ralph made a number
of mistakes, such as interpreting situations globally and behaving in ways
that didn't help him achieve his desired outcome. However, his in-session
SA performance improved to the point where he no longer needed remediation assistance from his CBASP therapist, Dr. Schultz—Ralph was
now able to self-correct his own mistakes when they occurred.

Our SA performance goal for you is the same. We want you to learn
to self-correct your mistakes until you no longer need assistance—you will

do it yourself. Once you can perform SA in the prescribed manner, you'll begin dealing with your problems one at a time, you'll stay focused in situations by interpreting them accurately, and you'll behave in ways that help you get what you want. Even in situations where you fail to achieve your desired outcome, you will be able to use SA to assess why the situation didn't work out and if the failure stemmed from something you did or didn't do or from someone else's behavior.

FIVE

The Interpersonal Discrimination Exercise

In this chapter, we introduce you to a second CBASP technique, the interpersonal discrimination exercise (IDE), that we will use to help you stop thinking in a global manner or resorting to the defeatist "it-doesn't-matter-what-I-do" approach to problem solving. Before describing this exercise, we need to consider the early lives of many chronically depressed adults. Understanding their early histories (which will probably ring a few bells for you) will help you see why the interpersonal discrimination exercise is a necessary part of CBASP treatment.

THE EARLY LIFE
OF CHRONICALLY DEPRESSED PATIENTS

A chronically depressed patient's early life experiences determine the expectations he or she brings to psychotherapy. Actually, this assumption about early life experiences affecting current expectations in therapy is true for all of us, regardless of the type of homelife we had—whether we describe our family environment as being negative, uneventful, or even positive. As noted in Chapter 2, many of our patients tell us that their early experiences were often negative. Parents, siblings, grandparents, aunts, uncles, or cousins were frequently the source of great distress, harm, and even severe trauma. Many of our patients commonly report negative experiences such as not having their emotional needs recognized or addressed, being physically neglected or sexually abused, or growing up around a parent or caretaker who was verbally abusive and denigrating.

Growing up in these negative environments leaves indelible scars that directly influence the way these adults now view themselves as well as other people—especially the psychotherapist. Early experiences of interpersonal trauma play out in psychotherapy in predictable ways because these patients have a predictable, global expectation: *The way things were for me in the past is the way things will be for me here.* Patients cannot rid themselves of the emotional pain associated with these early scars by telling themselves that their expectations are unreasonable. Something more is needed to heal the interpersonal wounds. That something is a "healing emotional experience" that occurs in a professional relationship with a caring human being who is personally involved with the patient *and* is respectful of the individual's personal space. The interpersonal discrimination exercise (IDE) is designed to provide the therapeutic emotional experience between therapist and patient that heals the wounds from early emotional trauma.

Thinking that negative interpersonal experiences from the past predict what will happen in the present with the therapist is another form of *global thinking.* Patients reflexively assume that people, in general, will behave in a manner similar to those significant others who inflicted the harm. The consequences of this global thinking are aversive emotional reactions—anxiety, shame, guilt, inadequacy, anger/rage, fear/terror—that make it impossible for these patients to tell the difference between those who will actually inflict harm and those who will not. Global thinking ensures that everyone gets lumped into the "heads up" category requiring chronic vigilance. The global thinking cycle is broken and a corrective emotional experience is put in its place by helping patients focus specifically on the patient–therapist relationship. How is this accomplished? It is accomplished by the IDE exercise described below.

SESSION TWO PREPARATIONS FOR DOING IDE WORK

We cannot know about the traumatic histories of our patients unless we ask about them—what it was like growing up in their families, and in what ways their significant others (parents, siblings, grandparents, and so on) influenced them to be the kind of persons they turned out to be. This information is obtained during the second session of CBASP, using a procedure called the "significant-other history."

Significant-Other History

You will be asked to provide your therapist with a list of up to seven significant others in your life. We can obtain more than enough information with this number. Now, what precisely do we mean by the label "significant others"? We mean, the major players in your life, not just good friends or acquaintances. Significant others are those people who have *left their stamp on you* in highly personal ways that influence the direction your life has taken. Without these people, you would not be the kind of person you are today.

A significant other can be an individual who has had either a *positive* or a *negative* (destructive) impact on you. One patient, Dan, after describing a father who always demanded perfection and who punished "every mistake [he] ever made," described the lasting impact of his father in the following way:

> "The stamp my father left on me was one of pervasive fear that I will make a mistake around somebody. I am *terrified* of making mistakes. The first thing I think about when I go to work every day is making a mistake. I even worry about making a mistake around my wife; even my children, for God's sake!"

Dan's father left a lasting impression on his son that has affected his entire life. Dan's fear of making mistakes is also going to influence the way he views his psychotherapist. He will most likely be afraid of making mistakes around the therapist. This fear of being punished if he makes a mistake will have to be addressed using the IDE. The example also illustrates what we said earlier about early life experiences with significant others affecting our expectations of what will happen to us in the therapy relationship.

Constructing the Transference Hypotheses

The psychological meaning of *transference* is that you and I take what we've learned in earlier relationships with significant others and transfer this interpersonal learning, in a global way, to present encounters. Another way to say the same thing is to say that the way we learned to feel, think, and behave toward significant others tends to be played out in the relationship with the therapist. Problems predictably arise in the therapeutic relationship when the patient's behavior toward the therapist is based not on what is really going on but on misperceptions caused by earlier learning. In these instances, the therapist is viewed as being someone he or she is not. Misperceptions in therapy frequently cause patients to think and act in a defeatist sort of way—"It doesn't matter what I do, nothing will work out for me." Defensive, avoidant, or angry reactions are often present on these occasions. In some cases, misperceptions of the CBASP therapist's behavior or motives have caused patients to leave treatment prematurely.

We know that our patients have valid reasons for expecting the worst from their therapists. It is no surprise that psychotherapy often begins on shaky ground—interpersonal trust is not yet in place. It is the therapist's "job" to replace these misperceptions with experiences that lead to interpersonal trust. One of the ways the CBASP therapist accomplishes this goal is by using the interpersonal discrimination exercise.

Let's return to Mary's and Ralph's experiences in CBASP therapy to see how the information from their significant-other history was used in the interpersonal discrimination exercise. The significant-other histories of these patients enabled their therapists to pinpoint potential interpersonal "hot spots" (transference issues) that might lead the patients to view their therapists in an unrealistic way. The material below is taken from the information we obtained from Mary's and Ralph's descriptions of their significant others. Each patient talked about seven significant individuals. Only three per patient are presented below.

Case 1 (Mary)

Mother. She was an alcoholic who was also chronically depressed. Mother committed suicide when I was 16. I had to run the household most of the time (wash, cook the meals, etc.) because she was intoxicated and wouldn't do anything. When I begged her to help me, she just shrugged me off. I never talked to her about anything. She never helped me do anything. I could never go to her and talk about my problems or anything else that I needed. *Mother's stamp on me:* No one can love me or be interested in anything I do or need.

Father. He was also alcoholic and was physically abusive when he was drunk. Dad was a binge drinker, and whenever I came home from school, I never knew whether he would be drunk or not. I never brought friends home or had them over. My household was always chaotic. My father never helped me do anything. I never learned anything from him. Drink, drink, drink was all he ever did. He was always telling me to do things for him—I was like his servant. *Father's stamp on me*: I grew up thinking I know nothing about life, I have no control over anything, and I have to take care of people. Everything is out of control, especially when it comes to men.

Older brother. He was five years older. Sam started demanding sex from me when I was eight years old. He would come to my bedroom at night when both of my parents were drunk. There was nothing I could do. He always threatened to "beat me up" if I ever told my parents. I never did. He left home when he was 16, so the sex stopped. I've hated him all my life. *Brother's stamp on me*: Guys will always take advantage of me. They'll never care about me. They'll just use me and dump me.

From Mary's significant-other history, it's clear that her male therapist begins treatment with "two strikes against him." The significant men in Mary's life have been unsavory and hurtful individuals. The therapist anticipates two potential interpersonal hot spots: One involves occasions when relational intimacy (for example, when the patient feels the vulnerability that comes from self-disclosure) is experienced, and the second is when Mary needs something from the therapist (such as emotional support). When such occasions arise during the session, it's easy to guess what Mary is likely to expect from the therapist: INTERPERSONAL TROUBLE AHEAD! What did this CBASP therapist do in anticipating these negative transference hot spots? He constructed two transference hypotheses from the significant-other history material and used them as a blueprint to administer the IDE. Note how the hypotheses constructed by Dr. Rowan are stated from Mary's point of view:

1. If I get close to Dr. Rowan, then he will abuse/hurt me, or I'll have to take care of him.
2. If I need something from Dr. Rowan, then he will be indifferent and not give me what I need.

Case 2 (Ralph)

Mother. She was very passive. I think she loved me, but she wasn't very demonstrative. She tried hard to be a wife and mother, but I don't think she was successful. She was totally dominated by my father. She made a lot of mistakes and often condemned herself for her foul-ups. *Mother's stamp on me*: Women can't be expected to do very much; they're kindhearted but pretty ineffective.

Father. He lorded it over my mother and me. He criticized my mother about everything. She could do nothing right. She just took his criticism and never protested. He used to tell me that I'd never do anything with my life! Dad always compared me to his brother's boy, whom he considered to be the "perfect son." He said that I would always be a failure. *Father's stamp on me*: He made me feel that no matter what I do, I'll always be incompetent and a failure.

Cousin. Jake did all the right things that I could never do. He was a straight-A student and a good athlete. He dated the most popular women. He did excellently in college, and I was always average. He's made a lot of money as a lawyer—my salary is modest compared to his. *Cousin's stamp on me*: I'll never measure up—I'm just a failure as a human being.

Ralph's therapist concluded from his significant-other history material that there would be two interpersonal hot-spot areas needing attention. One involved the area of relational intimacy (as was the case for Mary), and the other, that of making mistakes in front of the therapist. Ralph will have to learn that criticism and censure are not a part of the therapeutic relationship. He will also have to experience tangible assistance and support from his therapist whenever he talks about something he has done or when he makes a mistake. The transference hypotheses constructed on Ralph by Dr. Schultz were:

1. If I get close to Dr. Schultz, then he will remind me that I am an incompetent failure—I'll never measure up, in Dr. Schultz's eyes.
2. If I make a mistake (for example, miss an appointment, make mistakes on my SA, etc.), then Dr. Schultz will condemn me for my failure.

TREATING INTERPERSONAL HOT SPOTS WITH THE IDE

With these transference hypotheses "under their belts," CBASP therapists are equipped with the information that will enable them to soften the harsh learning histories patients bring to therapy. The harmful consequences that have always been present in these specific hot-spot situations will *not* occur in the therapy relationship. Hopefully, a healing emotional experience will take the place of these hurtful consequences, overthrowing global thinking and mending old interpersonal wounds.

Now we will consider two situations wherein Mary's and Ralph's therapists used the IDE to address interpersonal hot spots.

Case 1 (Mary)

Mary's therapist sensed that the content of her SA event (see Case 1 CSQ) involved a core hot spot: Mary needed help and emotional support to deal with an aggressive, insensitive neighbor. Using the second transference hypothesis as a blueprint (If I need something from Dr. Rowan, then he will be indifferent and not give me what I need), Dr. Rowan administered the IDE.

DR. ROWAN: This was a difficult situational analysis for you.

MARY: It was awful, but it's just like all the other things that happen to me.

DR. ROWAN: How would your mother have reacted if you had gone to her and asked her how you ought to handle this situation?

MARY: Good God! She would have told me to get lost! She would have probably been drunk. She couldn't have cared less about me or anything I might need or want. (*Mary is beginning to tear up.*)

DR. ROWAN: How would your father have reacted, had you asked for suggestions about dealing with this pushy neighbor?

MARY: He would have laughed me out of the room. Told me to go fix him some supper, or something like that. He always thought what I did was stupid. Had he been drunk, he might have slapped me. I would never have asked him something like this.

DR. ROWAN: I'm going to ask you something now, and I want you to think carefully before you answer. How did I react to you when you presented this very difficult situation to me?

MARY: (*after a minute or two*) You certainly didn't react the way my parents would have.

DR. ROWAN: How did I react to you?

MARY: You listened, you helped me fix the SA, and then you said I could do it whenever I was ready. I've never had anyone talk with me like this. (*Mary is crying now.*) You are kind to me even when I'm too scared to go out and put things into practice. I'm really not sure what to do with someone who treats me nice. It really feels weird, almost unnatural. Like, maybe I don't deserve such treatment.

DR. ROWAN: Sounds to me like you are experiencing something with me that is different and new for you. Sounds like it is different for you to experience respect and caring from a man. Am I right?

MARY: I don't know what to say. Yes, it is new and different. All I know is that it surely is nice. For some reason, I'm not afraid anymore.

DR. ROWAN: I want to ask you this. How would you compare my reaction to you with the way you described the likely reactions of your mother and father?

MARY: You are kind, and you listen to me. They never were. You are interested in helping me, and they never were. You seemed truly concerned about helping me work this situation out. I've never known anyone who was interested in helping me work out my problems. This was a very different experience for me. It feels different—it feels good, safe.

Case 2 (Ralph)

Ralph's situational behavior led to the attainment of his desired outcome (see Case 2 CSQ). But remember the last comment he made to Dr. Schultz at the end of the SA? He said, " . . . I'm still surprised when you tell me that I did a good job. I keep expecting you to lay in to me and tell me that I made a mistake and that I'm incompetent." We all know where this expectation comes from: Nothing he ever did with or for his father was right or good enough. The transference hypothesis (If I make a mistake, then Dr. Schultz will condemn me for my failure) comes to the forefront with Ralph's statement. This was an optimal time for Dr. Schultz to administer the IDE, and he did.

DR. SCHULTZ: Why did you say to me that you are surprised that I praised what you did in the situation and didn't criticize you for making a mistake?

RALPH: It's what I expect from everyone whenever I do something. I have this tape going on in my head that never shuts off: "You've screwed up, Ralph. You're a failure, Ralph. All you do is make mistakes, Ralph. You're incompetent, Ralph." The tape never stops when I'm around people.

DR. SCHULTZ: If you told your father about your success in this situation, how would he have reacted to you?

RALPH: He would call me a "stupid incompetent" for having forgotten the agreement I'd made with Phyllis. (*Ralph starts to become angry.*) Goddammit, he would have found ten things to find fault with about what I did. It would have been a nightmare. I would never tell him anything about something like this.

DR. SCHULTZ: How did I react to you?

RALPH: I couldn't believe what you said! You complimented me on how I handled the problem. Then you said that you might not have done as well. I've never known anyone to say this to me before. I still cannot believe you said this.

DR. SCHULTZ: Compare and contrast my reaction to you with the reaction you would expect from your father.

RALPH: It's like night and day.

DR. SCHULTZ: Try to be specific.

RALPH: All right. You were complimentary, supportive, and helpful. It makes me think I could tell you anything, and you wouldn't criticize me. It will take some getting used to on my part. I'm going to need a little time to think about this one.

DR. SCHULTZ: Take all the time you want.

The interpersonal discrimination exercise is a standardized procedure your therapist will use to compare his or her interpersonal behavior with that of your significant others. Discriminating between the therapist's behavior and that of harmful significant others often results in the healing of old interpersonal wounds. Healing usually takes place during difficult occasions when you are with someone who you feel cares about you, who stands clearly on your side, who is helpful without being invasive or judgmental, and who prevents you from overlooking the fact that there are essential differences between what he or she has done and what significant others have done to you in the past. The healing emotional experiences that result also enable you to gain control of your global thinking about people in general. Once your aversive reaction is decreased through beneficial experiences with your therapist, positive interpersonal encounters become possible. Your old conclusion that "It doesn't really matter what I do around others because things are going to turn out bad anyway" is exposed as untrue and discarded.

CONCLUSION

A successfully treated CBASP patient who stopped talking globally about her problems and no longer reacted to stress with the defeatist "It-doesn't-matter-what-I-do" response had this to say during the final session:

> "I don't know if you remember it or not, but the first time we met you told me that you had hope for me. I thought you were crazy. No one has ever had hope for me. Maybe I continued to come to therapy because of what you said; I'm not sure, but I surely am glad I hung in there. Now I have hope for myself. Not because it's a nice way to feel, but because I have proven to myself that I can control my life and the things that happen to me. I'm no longer helpless! When I get into situations now, the first thing I do is think about what I want. Then the next thing is to think about what I have to do to reach my goal. My entire life has become one of goal-setting. And you know, I'm producing what I want most of the time. I'm not helpless anymore!
>
> "Another thing I have realized is that I trust you. I've never been able to trust another human being in my life. What a wonderful feeling it is to be able to relax and trust you. I want to be able to stay in touch with you monthly. I will need you again or at least want to talk with you again. I'm launching out, and I think I'm ready."